FAST FACTS

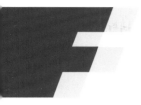

T5-AWF-306

Erectile Dysfunction
Second edition

Indispensable

Guides to

Clinical

Practice

Roger Kirby
Consultant Urologist,
St George's Hospital, London, UK

Simon Holmes
Consultant Urologist,
St Mary's Hospital, Portsmouth, UK

Culley Carson
Professor and Chief of Division of Urology,
The University of North Carolina,
Chapel Hill, North Carolina, USA

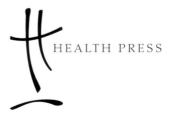

HEALTH PRESS

Oxford

Fast Facts – Erectile Dysfunction
First published as Male Erectile Dysfunction 1997
Second edition 1998
Reprinted 1999

Elizabeth House, Queen Street,
Abingdon, Oxford, UK OX14 3JR

Tel: +44 (0)1235 523233
Fax: +44 (0)1235 523238

Fast Facts is a trademark of Health Press Limited.

A CIP catalogue record for this title is available from
the British Library.

ISBN 1-899541-47-0

Library of Congress
Cataloging-in-Publication Data

Kirby, R. (Roger)
Fast Facts – Erectile Dysfunction/
Roger Kirby, Simon Holmes,
Culley Carson

Illustrated by Dee McLean,
MeDee Art, London, UK

Printed by Sterling Press, Wellingborough, UK.

Glossary

Corpora cavernosa: paired columns of erectile tissue in the penis

cGMP: cyclic guanosine monophosphate, the second messenger molecule that facilitates the vasodilatation that leads to erection

Detumescence: loss of turgidity and erection, usually caused by active sympathetic stimulation

ED: erectile dysfunction

Intracavernosal self-injection: technique in which the patient injects vasoactive drugs into his corpora cavernosa

MUSE®: medicated urethral system for erection

NO: nitric oxide, a neurotransmitter that produces an erection

Organic erectile dysfunction: erectile dysfunction caused by the failure of one or more of the essential stages in penile erection, namely the arterial blood supply, venous occlusion or neurological control

PDE 5: phosphodiesterase type 5, the substance that breaks down cGMP, resulting in detumescence

PGE_1: prostaglandin E_1, a neurotransmitter resulting in erection

Priapism: an erection that lasts for more than 4 hours

Psychogenic erectile dysfunction: erectile dysfunction caused by higher brain centre influences in the presence of a normal erectile mechanism

Spinal erection centre: an area in the spinal cord through which the spinal erection reflex passes, and which is under neural control from higher brain centres

Tumescence: vasodilatation in the corpora cavernosa resulting in erection

Vasoactive agents: drugs that have a dilatory effect on blood vessels

Veno-occlusive mechanism: the mechanism by which the venous drainage of the erectile tissues is occluded to allow filling of the lacunar spaces resulting in penile turgidity

VED: vacuum erection device

VIP: vasoactive intestinal polypeptide

Introduction

A man who is unable to develop or sustain an erection sufficient for penetrative sexual intercourse is usually labelled 'impotent' – a word that not only has pejorative implications, but also takes little account of the complex process of male sexual function. Erectile dysfunction (ED) is now the preferred term. The concerned clinician will consider a patient's inability to develop an erect penis within a given psychological and behavioural context, and recognize that although isolated ED is by far the most common problem, reduced libido and impaired orgasmic or ejaculatory capacity may also coexist to varying degrees, each contributing to the patient's loss of confidence and sense of inadequacy. Recently there has been a surge of interest in the causes of, and remedies for, ED.

Erectile dysfunction affects many millions of men (and it is also becoming appreciated that some women suffer from significant sexual dysfunction), and although it may not mean total loss of sexual satisfaction for some, for most it creates mental stress and anxiety that adversely affects their personal relationships and quality of life. It is often assumed to be a natural part of ageing, and therefore a misfortune which simply has to be accepted and borne stoically. This assumption is not, however, always correct. Erectile dysfunction may occur as a result of a specific illness (e.g. diabetes) or the medical treatment of others (e.g. hypertension) resulting in additional anxiety, loss of confidence and depression. Accurate assessment requires recognition by both patient and doctor that the problem is only part of overall male sexual dysfunction: both psychological and organic components need to be considered, along with personal circumstances. Relationship difficulties also need to be taken into account and, in this respect, the family physician is well placed to play an important role.

Since ED is never life-threatening, patient preference must always be paramount in decisions relating to diagnosis and treatment. The Process of Care Model identifies the following steps in the management of this prevalent condition:

- problem identification
- patient assessment and diagnosis
- modification of reversible causes
- first-, second- and third-line treatment interventions.

In most men, ED can now be accurately diagnosed and effectively treated using a rapidly increasing number of well-tolerated and effective therapeutic options. However, many of these advances are still incompletely understood by patients and healthcare professionals alike, and the condition can go undiagnosed and untreated for long periods, often becoming compounded by its psychological sequelae.

It is hoped that the information contained in this second edition of *Fast Facts – Erectile Dysfunction* will help point the way towards an improved quality of life for the many sufferers of ED and their partners.

CHAPTER 1

Epidemiology and pathophysiology

Epidemiology

Precise figures for the prevalence of erectile dysfunction (ED) in male populations around the world are difficult to obtain. However, data from a number of US and UK studies are similar and these figures are regarded as the best estimate. The prevalence of complete ED is estimated to be approximately 5% among 40-year-olds, 10% among men in their 60s, 15% in their 70s and 30–40% in their 80s (Figure 1.1). From these figures it has been estimated that there may be 20 million men in the USA, and perhaps as many in Europe, who have significant problems with erectile function.

Risk factors for erectile dysfunction. Apart from age, other important risk factors for ED include diabetes mellitus, hypertension, hyperlipidaemia, depression and smoking. Obesity, over-consumption of alcohol and lack of regular exercise may also contribute to the problem. Men with

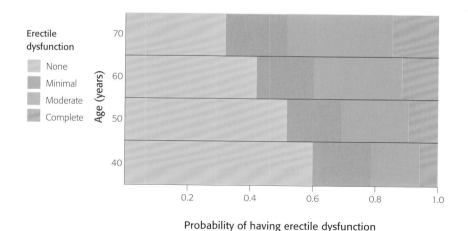

Figure 1.1 Relationship between age and the probablity of erectile dysfunction. Data from the Massachusetts Male Aging Study (Feldman et al. *J Urol* 1994;150:54–61).

hypothyroidism and chronic renal failure are prone to ED, and hypogonadism and hyperprolactinaemia are also important causes of endocrine-associated erectile difficulties.

Anatomy and physiology of the normal erection

The penis consists of three cylindrical columns of tissue surrounded by a sturdy fascial layer (Buck's fascia), subcutaneous tissue and skin (Figure 1.2). Paired cylinders of erectile tissue, the corpora cavernosa, run the length of the penis, surrounded by a thick, non-expansile fibrous envelope, the tunica albuginea. Each corporal body communicates with the other through the medial septum that separates them. The erectile tissue itself is composed of a distensible lattice of blood sinusoids surrounded by trabeculae of smooth muscle, which control the sinusoidal blood capacity. The corpus spongiosum of the penis surrounds the urethra and expands to form the sensitive glans penis; it contains similar erectile tissue and is enclosed within the very thin tunica albuginea.

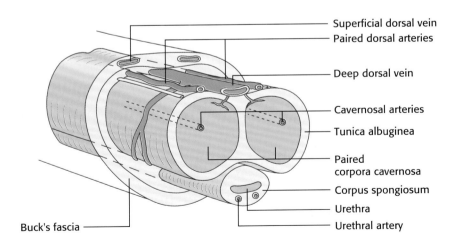

Figure 1.2 Cross-sectional anatomy of the penis.

Vascular supply. The arterial blood flow to the penis (Figure 1.3) originates from the internal iliac arteries via the internal pudendal arteries. The internal pudendal arteries terminate as the penile arteries, which divide to form:
- the dorsal artery
- the cavernosal artery, which runs down the centre of each corpus cavernosum
- the bulbo-urethral artery, which supplies the corpus spongiosum.

The cavernosal artery gives off numerous branches along its length, called helicine arteries, which supply blood to the sinusoids of the erectile tissue.

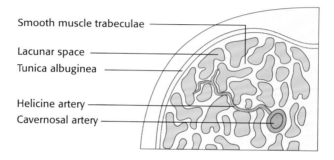

Smooth muscle trabeculae

Lacunar space
Tunica albuginea

Helicine artery
Cavernosal artery

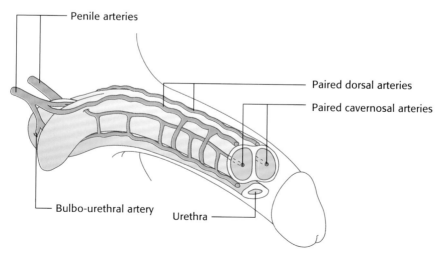

Penile arteries

Paired dorsal arteries

Paired cavernosal arteries

Bulbo-urethral artery   Urethra

Figure 1.3 Arterial blood supply of the penis and corpora cavernosa.

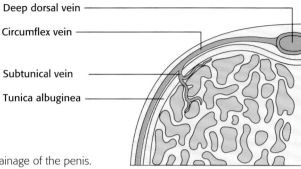

Deep dorsal vein

Circumflex vein

Subtunical vein

Tunica albuginea

Figure 1.4 Venous drainage of the penis.

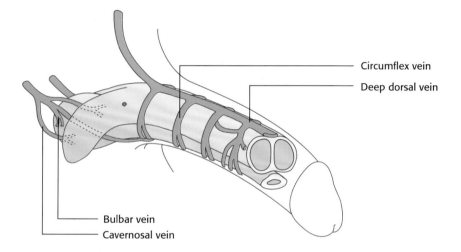

Circumflex vein

Deep dorsal vein

Bulbar vein

Cavernosal vein

The venous drainage system collects blood from the sinusoids that run obliquely under the tunica albuginea, before exiting through the tunica as emissary veins to collect in the deep dorsal vein of the penis. The deep dorsal vein runs up the dorsal surface of the penis and joins the periprostatic venous complex (Figure 1.4). Cavernosal veins drain the proximal portions of the corpora.

Peripheral nerve supply. The mechanism of erection is controlled by the autonomic nervous system. Parasympathetic nerves from S2–4 are the principle mediators of erection, while sympathetic nerves from T11–L2 control ejaculation and detumescence. These autonomic fibres unite in the pelvic plexus to form the cavernous nerves, which run down behind the prostate and into the base of the penis. These nerves and the pelvic plexus itself are susceptible to damage from any form of pelvic surgery.

The pelvic nerves contain sensory and motor elements that form a reflex arc through the spinal cord, in an area known as the spinal erection centre. A 'reflex' erection therefore occurs as a direct result of stimulation of the penis, and can even occur in patients who have suffered a suprasacral spinal cord transection.

Mechanism of erection

Neuroendocrine messages from the brain (due to either audiovisual stimuli or fantasy), either with or without tactile stimulation of the penis, activate the autonomic nuclei of the spinal erection centre, which send messages to the erectile tissue of the corpora cavernosa via the cavernosal nerves. These result in:

- dilatation of the cavernosal and helicine arteries, increasing blood flow into the lacunar spaces
- relaxation of cavernosal smooth muscle, opening the vascular lacunar space
- expansion of the lacunar spaces against the tunica albuginea, compressing the obliquely running subtunical venous drainage channels, decreasing venous outflow and producing a rigid erection; this is the veno-occlusive mechanism (Figure 1.5).

Detumescence. Reversal of these events causes detumescence, and is caused by increased sympathetic vasoconstrictor activity and the enzymatic breakdown of cyclic guanosine monophosphate (cGMP) by phosphodiesterase type 5 (PDE 5). This occurs naturally after orgasm and ejaculation, both of which are also mediated by the sympathetic nervous system.

Molecular basis of erection

The key modulator of erection is the tone of the smooth muscle walls of the helicine arteries and the trabecular spaces. This is controlled by the level of intracellular calcium in the smooth muscle cells. A number of neurotransmitters and endothelium-derived factors are able to influence intracellular calcium and thereby alter the balance between penile flaccidity and erection (Figure 1.6).

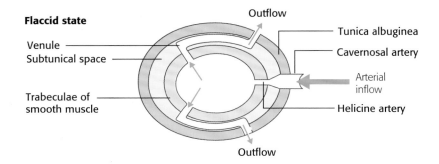

Flaccid state

Venule
Subtunical space
Trabeculae of
smooth muscle

Outflow
Tunica albuginea
Cavernosal artery
Arterial
inflow
Helicine artery
Outflow

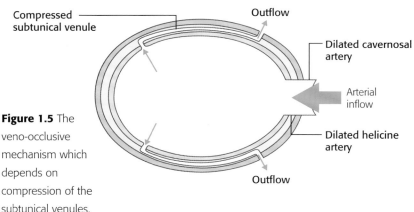

Erect state

Compressed
subtunical venule

Outflow
Dilated cavernosal
artery
Arterial
inflow
Dilated helicine
artery
Outflow

Figure 1.5 The veno-occlusive mechanism which depends on compression of the subtunical venules.

Smooth muscle relaxation. Nitric oxide (NO) is the most important neurotransmitter in this system. Produced from L-arginine by the enzyme nitric oxide synthase, NO diffuses into the smooth muscle cells, where it activates a guanylate cyclase second messenger system. Guanylate cyclase converts guanosine triphosphate (GTP) into cGMP. This then activates the sodium pump system and opens potassium channels, causing a decrease in intracellular calcium. The effect of cGMP is ended by enzymatic breakdown – the enzyme involved, PDE 5, exists principally in the corpora cavernosa.

Other vasodilator mechanisms exist, including ones involving vasoactive intestinal polypeptide (VIP) and prostaglandin E_1 (PGE_1), both of which act through the adenylate cyclase system. Vasoactive intestinal polypeptide and PGE_1 molecules stimulate the production of cyclic adenosine monophosphate (cAMP) from adenosine triphosphate (ATP).

Like cGMP, cAMP reduces intracellular calcium and thereby induces smooth muscle relaxation.

Smooth muscle contraction. The vasoconstrictor noradrenaline (NA) counterbalances the smooth muscle relaxation mechanisms. Noradrenaline is released from sympathetic nerve terminals within the corpora, and diffuses across the synaptic gap. It activates α_1-adrenoceptors on the cell membranes of smooth muscle cells. These α_1-adrenoceptors are linked to second messenger pathways that raise intracellular calcium, either by facilitating entry of calcium from the extracellular compartment, or by releasing calcium from intracellular organelles. A number of other molecules that increase intracellular calcium, such as endothelin-1 and prostaglandin F_2, are probably equally involved in the maintenance of flaccidity. Increased free calcium levels within the smooth muscle cells of the helicine arteries and the trabecular smooth muscle cells activate the contractile mechanism by which actin and myosin molecules slide over each other and form new cross

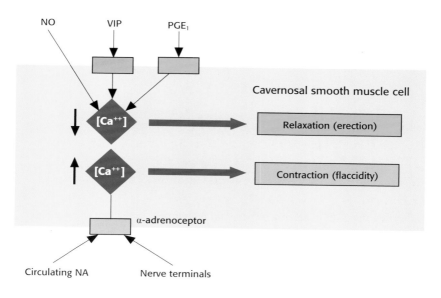

PGE₁   Prostaglandin E₁
VIP   Vasoactive intestinal polypeptide
NO   Nitric oxide
NA   Noradrenaline

Figure 1.6 Factors that influence balance between erection and flaccidity.

bridges. Once these are created, a tonic contractile state can be maintained with almost zero energy consumption.

Neural influence

A number of neural pathways to and from the brain influence and sometimes initiate an erectile response. A 'psychogenic' erection occurs as a result of audiovisual stimuli or sexual fantasy via signals from the brain to the spinal erection centre activating the erectile process (Figure 1.7). However, these pathways can also act to inhibit the same process, giving

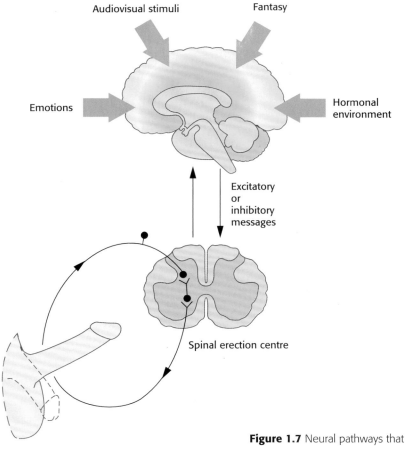

Audiovisual stimuli

Fantasy

Emotions

Hormonal environment

Excitatory or inhibitory messages

Spinal erection centre

Tumescence

Figure 1.7 Neural pathways that influence the erectile response.

rise to psychogenic ED. Several areas in the brain are important in this respect. One is the paraventricular nucleus of the hypothalamus, where dopamine is the key neurotransmitter mediating co-ordination of neuronal activity.

Causes of erectile dysfunction

The causes of ED (Table 1.1) may be due to changes in the:

- CNS, at the level of either the brain or the spinal cord

TABLE 1.1

Causes of erectile dysfunction

Psychogenic

- Anxiety
- Loss of attraction
- Relationship difficulties
- Stress

Psychiatric

- Depression

Neurogenic

- Trauma
- Myelodysplasia (spina bifida)
- Intervertebral disc lesion
- Multiple sclerosis
- Diabetes mellitus
- Alcohol
- Pelvic surgery

Endocrine

- Hormonal deficiency – low testosterone; raised sex hormone-binding globulin; high prolactin

Arteriogenic

- Hypertension
- Smoking
- Diabetes mellitus
- Hyperlipidaemia
- Peripheral vascular disease

Venous

- Functional impairment of the veno-occlusive mechanism

Drugs

- Central and/or direct effect, most commonly implicated antihypertensives, antidepressants and luteinizing hormone-releasing hormone analogues

These conditions are not mutually exclusive, many cases of erectile dysfunction are multifactorial

- peripheral nervous system, usually due to diabetes mellitus, trauma or surgical injury
- corpora cavernosa, as in Peyronie's disease
- vascular system – either arterial insufficiency or a disorder of the veno-occlusive mechanism
- endocrine system – reduced testosterone or increased prolactin.

Although it was originally believed that psychogenic problems were the predominant cause of ED, it has now been shown that organic causes are more common, particularly in middle-aged and older men presenting to an ED clinic. In one study, for example, 11% of new patients attending an ED clinic were found to have undiagnosed diabetes and more than half had vascular problems. Almost all patients, however, have some psychogenic component to their symptoms.

CHAPTER 2

Diagnosis

A full history and thorough clinical examination of the patient are needed to:
- help elucidate the cause of ED
- determine whether the problem is psychogenic or organic in origin
- identify any clinical signs of the known risk factors.

It should be borne in mind that ED can be an early symptom of a more systemic condition, such as diabetes mellitus or vascular disease.

Referral to an appropriate physician may be necessary if there is evidence of:
- significant peripheral vascular disease
- an organic cause of ED in a young man (e.g. depression)
- hypogonadism in a young man.

Findings from the history and examination of the patient can be supplemented by investigations to identify the cause of erectile failure. Investigations can be used to:
- confirm the associated underlying condition (e.g. diabetes mellitus)
- give a differential diagnosis of specific causes of ED.

History

The clinical history has several purposes:
- to confirm that the patient is suffering from ED
- to assess the severity of the condition
- to identify a possible underlying aetiology.

The initial aim, therefore, is to determine whether the problem is one of ED and whether or not this is accompanied by ejaculatory dysfunction, diminished libido or loss of orgasm.

The terminology associated with ED is often confused, and men's expectations of their sexual function may be unrealistic. The severity of the problem can often be assessed by asking simple questions such as, 'when did you last have successful sexual intercourse?' and 'how frequently do you have problems with your erection?'

Many doctor/patient consultations about ED are initiated by the doctor. The patient may present with an unrelated problem and only when

TABLE 2.1

Medical conditions associated with ED

	Incidence (%)
Depression	70
Diabetes mellitus	50
Heart disease	40
Hypertension	15

questioned more closely will he reveal his true concerns. Likewise, there are a number of medical conditions that are now well recognized as being associated with ED (Table 2.1).

Once the degree of ED has been established, tactful enquiries can be made about a possible aetiology. The aim of the subsequent discussion is to differentiate between obvious psychological causes and organic causes of the problem. Many men have a combination of causes, however, and the history will contain both organic and psychogenic elements. Topics to include in discussions with patients include:

- the patient's sexual development
- the patient and his partner's attitude to the problem
- the presence of any obvious stress factors, such as marital problems, financial concerns, sexual inhibitions
- medical and drug history.

The diagnosis of psychogenic and/or organic causes is based on a number of factors.

Psychogenic erectile dysfunction. The association between anxiety and ED should be established. A psychological element should be suspected in a patient who obtains an erection during foreplay or self-stimulation, but fails or fears failure on penetration. Performance anxiety is almost universal in men with a purely psychogenic problem. In these men, early morning and nocturnal erections are often preserved (Table 2.2). Onset of dysfunction is usually sudden and may relate to a specific occasion or life event. A more detailed psychosexual history, exploring sources of anxiety, guilt, relationship difficulties or depression should be obtained.

TABLE 2.2

Differential diagnosis of psychogenic and organic ED

Psychogenic	Organic
● Sudden onset	● Gradual onset
● Specific situation	● All circumstances
● Normal nocturnal and early morning erections	● Absent nocturnal and early morning erections
● Relationship problems	● Normal libido and ejaculation
● Problems during sexual development	● Normal sexual development

Organic erectile dysfunction is characterized by a progressive loss of erectile function with a gradual loss of sustainable erectile rigidity, often combined with the loss of early morning and nocturnal erections (Table 2.2). Both libido and ejaculatory function are usually maintained. The International Index of Erectile Function (IIEF), devised by Rosen and colleagues, allows a more objective assessment of the problem, in the same way that symptom scores are used in the evaluation of men suffering from prostate disorders (Table 2.3). The scoring system provides a method of measuring a patient's progress from an initial 'benchmark' level.

Concomitant medication. A detailed medical history should be taken to check for the presence of any recognized risk factors. In particular, careful enquiry should be made about current medications, as well as the use of recreational drugs. A number of these may cause or contribute to ED (Table 2.4). For example, antihypertensive agents, such as β-blockers and diuretics, are associated with ED. In such cases it may be worthwhile changing the patient's medication to an α-adrenoceptor antagonist such as doxazosin or terazosin. Because of the vasodilatory effects of this class of drug, they may be mildly beneficial in ED.

Erectile dysfunction is a common complication of antidepressant therapy with either monoamine oxidase inhibitors or tricyclic antidepressants. Selective serotonin re-uptake inhibitors may cause both ED and retarded ejaculation.

TABLE 2.3

The IIEF symptom score system devised for patients with ED*

Over the past 4 weeks:

1 How often were you able to get an erection during sexual activity?

2 When you had erections with sexual stimulation, how often were your erections hard enough for penetration?

0 = No sexual activity
1 = Almost never/never
2 = A few times (much less than half the time)
3 = Sometimes (about half the time)
4 = Most times (much more than half the time)
5 = Almost always/always

3 When you attempted sexual intercourse, how often were you able to penetrate (enter) your partner?

4 During sexual intercourse, how often were you able to maintain your erection after you had penetrated (entered) your partner?

0 = Did not attempt intercourse
1 = Almost never/never
2 = A few times (much less than half the time)
3 = Sometimes (about half the time)
4 = Most times (much more than half the time)
5 = Almost always/always

5 During sexual intercourse, how difficult was it to maintain your erection to completion of intercourse?

0 = Did not attempt intercourse
1 = Extremely difficult
2 = Very difficult
3 = Difficult
4 = Slightly difficult
5 = Not difficult

6 How many times have you attempted sexual intercourse?

0 = No attempts
1 = 1–2 attempts
2 = 3–4 attempts
3 = 5–6 attempts
4 = 7–10 attempts
5 = 11+ attempts

7 When you attempted sexual intercourse, how often was it satisfactory for you?

0 = Did not attempt intercourse
1 = Almost never/never
2 = A few times (much less than half the time)
3 = Sometimes (about half the time)
4 = Most times (much more than half the time)
5 = Almost always/always

8	How much have you enjoyed sexual intercourse?	0 = No intercourse

0 = No intercourse
1 = No enjoyment
2 = Not very enjoyable
3 = Fairly enjoyable
4 = Highly enjoyable
5 = Very highly enjoyable

8 How much have you enjoyed sexual intercourse?

0 = No intercourse
1 = No enjoyment
2 = Not very enjoyable
3 = Fairly enjoyable
4 = Highly enjoyable
5 = Very highly enjoyable

9 When you had sexual stimulation or intercourse, how often did you ejaculate?

10 When you had sexual stimulation or intercourse, how often did you have the feeling of orgasm or climax?

0 = No sexual stimulation/intercourse
1 = Almost never/never
2 = A few times (much less than half the time)
3 = Sometimes (about half the time)
4 = Most times (much more than half the time)
5 = Almost always/always

11 How often have you felt sexual desire?

1 = Almost never/never
2 = A few times (much less than half the time)
3 = Sometimes (about half the time)
4 = Most times (much more than half the time)
5 = Almost always/always

12 How would you rate your level of sexual desire?

1 = Very low/none at all
2 = Low
3 = Moderate
4 = High
5 = Very high

13 How satisfied have you been with your overall sex life?

14 How satisfied have you been with your sexual relationship with your partner?

1 = Very dissatisfied
2 = Moderately dissatisfied
3 = About equally satisfied and dissatisfied
4 = Moderately satisfied
5 = Very satisfied

15 How do you rate your confidence that you could get and keep an erection?

1 = Very low
2 = Low
3 = Moderate
4 = High
5 = Very high

*Adapted with permission from Rosen et al. *Urology* 1997;49:822–830.

TABLE 2.4

Medications associated with ED

Major tranquillizers

- Phenothiazines
  (e.g. fluphenazine,
  chlorpromazine, promazine,
  mesoridazine)
- Butyrophenones
  (e.g. haloperidol)
- Thiozanthines (e.g. thiothixine,
  chorprothixene)

Anticholinergics

- Atropine
- Propantheline
- Benztrophine
- Dimenhydrinate
- Diphenhydramine

Luteinizing hormone-releasing hormone analogues

Antiandrogens

Antihypertensives

- Diuretics (e.g. thiazides,
  spironolactone)
- Vasodilators (e.g. hydralazine)
- Central sympatholytics
  (e.g. methyldopa, clonidine,
  reserpine)
- Ganglion blockers
  (e.g. guanethidine, bethanidine)
- β-blockers (e.g. propanolol,
  metoprolol, atenolol)
- ACE inhibitors (e.g. enalapril)
- Calcium channel blockers
  (e.g. nifedipine)

Antidepressants

- Tricyclics (e.g. nortryptyline,
  amitriptyline, desipramine,
  doxepin)
- Monoamine oxidase inhibitors
  (e.g. isocarboazide, phenelzine,
  tranylcypromine, pargylene,
  procarbine)

Anxiolytics

- Benzodiazepines
  (e.g. chlordiazepoxide,
  diazepam, chorazepate)

Psychotropic drugs

- Alcohol
- Marijuana
- Amphetamines
- Barbiturates
- Nicotine
- Opiates

Miscellaneous

- Cimetidine
- Clofibrate
- Digoxin
- Oestrogens
- Indomethacin
- Others

Physical examination

The examination of a man with ED will be directed, to a certain extent, by knowledge gained from his history. However, it is important to assess the external genitalia, the endocrine and vascular systems, and the prostate gland in most patients (Figure 2.1).

The presence, location and size of the testes, together with an assessment of secondary sexual characteristics will usually be enough to identify obvious hypogonadism.

Vascular assessment should include measurement of blood pressure, cardiac status and lower extremity pulses; a palpable aortic aneurysm should be sought. The penis should be carefully palpated to exclude the presence of fibrous Peyronie's plaques.

The prostate should be the same rubbery consistency as the tip of the nose. The presence of induration, or a palpable nodule, should raise the suspicion of prostate cancer. Serum levels of prostate-specific antigen (PSA) should be obtained and, if this is elevated in relation to the patient's age, he should be referred for transrectal ultrasound (TRUS) guided biopsy.

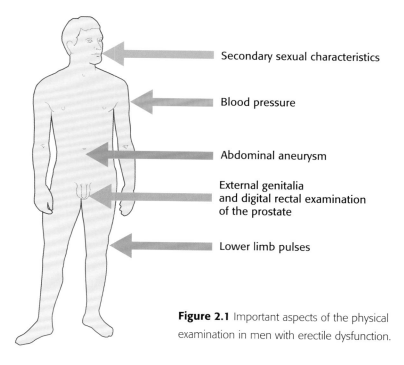

Secondary sexual characteristics

Blood pressure

Abdominal aneurysm

External genitalia
and digital rectal examination
of the prostate

Lower limb pulses

Figure 2.1 Important aspects of the physical examination in men with erectile dysfunction.

Clinical investigations

The degree to which men should undergo clinical investigation depends on the history of the problem, the experience of the physician, and the wishes of the patient. Diabetes mellitus should be excluded by testing the urine and blood for excess glucose; this is the only essential investigation. In some circumstances, treatment may then be initiated without further investigation. With oral treatments for ED now available, this may become standard practice. If the initial treatment is not successful, refer the patient for further investigations. These can be classed as general or specialized (Table 2.5).

General investigations include serum concentrations of testosterone, sex hormone-binding globulin (SHBG), prolactin, thyroid hormones, creatinine, PSA and fasting lipid levels. Special investigations are not always required, but may be necessary if patients fail to respond to minimally invasive treatments, before other options can be explored. Unless the problem is obviously psychogenic, most patients will have a trial injection of an intracavernosal vasoactive agent (see page 38) and their response assessed.

Specialized investigations need only be performed when a detailed knowledge of the cause of ED is required, and the patient and his partner have expressed an interest in pursuing corrective therapy.

TABLE 2.5

Clinical investigations for ED

Essential	General	Specialized
• Urine dipstick	• Serum testosterone	• Nocturnal penile tumescence testing
• Serum glucose	• Sex hormone-binding globulin	• Colour Doppler imaging
	• Prolactin	• Pharmaco-cavernosography
	• Creatinine	• Pharmaco-arteriography
	• Thyroid hormones	
	• Fasting lipid profile	
	• PSA	

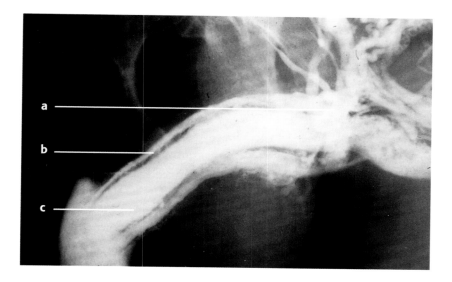

Figure 2.2 Venous leakage is occurring through the dorsal vein and into the retropubic venous plexus during pharmacocavernosography: (a) retropubic venous plexus; (b) dorsal vein; (c) corpus cavernosum.

Nocturnal penile tumescence testing. The presence of nocturnal erections, which is used to differentiate psychogenic from organic impotence, can be detected using devices placed around the penis during sleep. This is known as nocturnal penile tumescence (NPT) testing. The Snap-Gauge band and Rigiscan device are designed to be used at home and record the occurrence of nocturnal erections. Determining the presence or absence of nocturnal erections can also help treatment decisions.

Colour Doppler imaging provides information about penile haemodynamics after maximal smooth muscle relaxation has been induced with a vasoactive agent. Its aim is to distinguish arterial insufficiency from other causes of erectile failure. The velocity of blood in the cavernosal artery in the dynamic state can be measured during systole and diastole, and organic impotence can be differentiated from psychogenic impotence. It can also suggest the presence of a venous leak, although further studies are necessary to confirm this.

Pharmacocavernosography. Failure of the veno-occlusive mechanism to provide adequate venous outflow resistance can be demonstrated by pharmacocavernosography. This measures the blood flow required to maintain a pharmacologically stimulated erection. Contrast medium injected into the corpora will identify the location of any leak, which often originates in the deep dorsal vein of the penis (Figure 2.2), but may also be present in less accessible cavernosal veins.

Pharmaco-arteriography. In young men with ED caused by pelvic or perineal trauma, pudendal arteriography before and after a pharmacologically stimulated erection will identify those requiring arterial bypass.

CHAPTER 3

Treatment options

The treatment options for psychogenic and organic ED depend on the experience of the clinician, the wishes of the patient and the facilities that are available (Table 3.1). An approach to the treatment and management of ED is summarized in Figure 3.1.

TABLE 3.1

Treatment options in psychogenic and organic ED

Psychogenic	Organic
● Psychosexual therapy	● Oral pharmacological agents
● Oral pharmacological agents	● Intraurethral therapy
● Intraurethral therapy	● Intracavernosal therapy
● Intracavernosal therapy	● Vacuum devices
	● Androgen replacement therapy
	● Surgery

Psychogenic erectile dysfunction

Erections are often stimulated by audiovisual stimuli or fantasy; in the same way, however, other CNS signals can inhibit the erectile response. Inhibitory messages from the brain, acting on the spinal erection centre, prevent not only the 'psychogenic' erection, but also the 'reflex' erection by modulating the normal reflex arc. The inhibitory influence of the brain on erectile function may also be caused by an increased sympathetic outflow and the release of systemic catecholamines, which are known to inhibit the erectile response and cause detumescence (Figure 3.2).

Psychogenic ED can be caused by a number of problems, such as performance anxiety, guilt, depression, relationship problems, or by fear and personal anxiety (Figure 3.3). Performance anxiety is an especially common cause of erectile problems and may be self-perpetuating, with any subsequent attempts at sexual contact being burdened by a 'fear of failure' that only serves to exacerbate the problem. Concerns over whether an

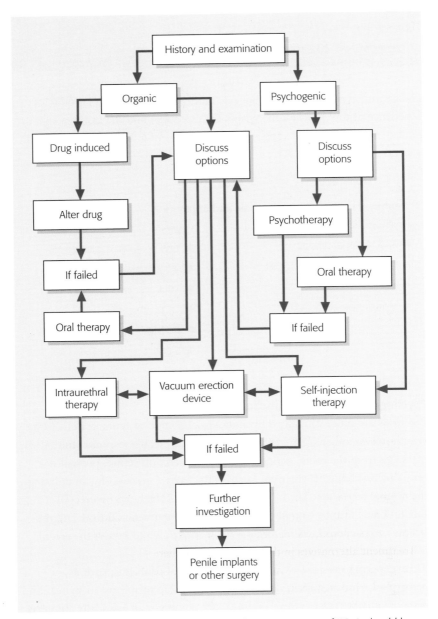

Figure 3.1 Goal-oriented treatment options in the management of ED. It should be remembered that, at any stage, the patient may decide to opt out of therapy and simply accept their condition.

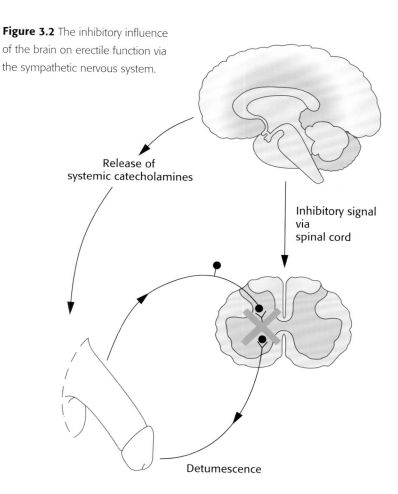

Figure 3.2 The inhibitory influence of the brain on erectile function via the sympathetic nervous system.

Release of
systemic catecholamines

Inhibitory signal
via
spinal cord

Detumescence

adequate and sustainable erection will develop, lead to 'spectatoring', (i.e. anxious scrutiny of a developing erection), which only serves to inhibit normal sexual responses further.

Treatment alternatives in this situation are either:

- to identify the source of anxiety, guilt or depression and provide a psychological treatment
- to initiate a physical (drug) treatment that overcomes the specific problem of ED.

Once a patient can obtain an erection 'on-demand' from a physical therapy, he may overcome performance anxiety himself.

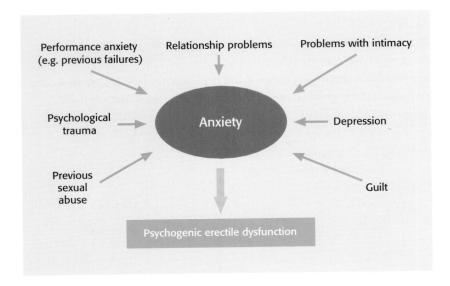

Figure 3.3 Causes of psychogenic erectile dysfunction.

Psychosexual therapy. Treatment for psychogenic ED cannot be standardized because the source of anxiety varies between patients. Relationship difficulties, depression, guilt, problems with intimacy and lack of sexual experience may all increase anxiety and/or conflict that may be manifested as ED.

Psychosexual treatments range from simple sex education through improved partner communication to cognitive and behavioural therapy. The onus is on the counsellor to identify the source of anxiety and select an appropriate therapy. Sex education usually involves correction of misinformation and ignorance about normal sexual practice. Improving partner communication may allow partners to overcome their embarrassment about sexual matters and express their sexual needs and desires.

Modern sex therapy owes much to the contribution of Masters and Johnson. They described a treatment programme involving a combination of behavioural and psychosexual elements, and reported a 70% success rate after 5 years of follow up. Today, therapy is more behaviour-based and aims to reduce performance anxiety via a programmed relearning of a couple's sexual behaviour. Often, this is achieved by gradually increasing a couple's repertoire of sexual activities that do not depend on maintaining a full erection, until full confidence is restored.

The drawback to these types of therapy is that they are expensive in terms of time and resources. They also usually require the presence and co-operation of the sexual partner, though initial individual consultations often help identify relationship problems and expectations. Few long-term studies have assessed the eventual outcomes of these treatments, though there appears to be a substantial recurrence rate after therapy. Many couples, however, derive genuine benefit from this approach, which can also be combined with oral pharmacological therapy.

Physical therapies.
Oral pharmacological agents. Although oral drug therapies have historically had a very limited role in the treatment of men with ED, it now seems that well-tolerated and successful treatment is possible. Oral therapy can be taken either as a course that gradually restores erectile function, or intermittently as an 'on-demand' drug.

The 'on-demand' concept is the basis of other physical treatments such as intracavernosal and intraurethral drugs, and vacuum devices. However, the rates of discontinuation with these treatment alternatives are high due to side-effects, dislike of needles and unwillingness of the partner to participate. This has provided the stimulus for the development of effective oral drugs – many are under development, awaiting approval or have recently been released. Because many of these agents have different sites of action, it is anticipated that drug combinations may act synergistically, though at present this remains a theoretical observation.

Intraurethral therapy. These treatments deliver vasoactive drugs to the corpora cavernosa via the urethral mucosa. The urethra has a rich submucosal blood supply that communicates with the corpora cavernosa through the corpus spongiosum, allowing delivery of vasoactive drugs to the corporal bodies. Therapeutic drug levels can be achieved in men with both psychogenic and organic ED.

Intracavernosal therapy. Erections can be stimulated pharmacologically using a vasoactive drug; this can be used to treat psychogenic ED enabling intercourse to take place and, with time, may eradicate the 'fear of failure' anxiety associated with the condition. Reliance on the drug to produce a satisfactory erection should then diminish, until eventually it is no longer required.

Combined psychogenic/organic erectile dysfunction

A large proportion of patients have a combination of psychogenic and organic ED. Erectile failure resulting from a developing organic problem may provoke the onset of a psychogenic effect once the patient develops the 'fear of failure' on sexual contact. To treat these men holistically, the family physician and psychotherapist may need to collaborate and combine counselling with a physical therapy, such as an oral pharmacological agent.

Organic erectile dysfunction

Organic ED will only respond to physical therapy. Treatment can be either cause-specific and aim to correct an identifiable abnormality, or general and aim to provide an erectile response regardless of underlying cause.

Androgen replacement therapy for hypogonadal men. Male hypogonadism, leading to testosterone deficiency and impotence, can have a number of causes (Table 3.2). Regardless of aetiology, the aim of androgen replacement therapy is to maintain secondary sexual characteristics and sexual behaviour. All hormone substitution therapy aims to achieve physiological serum concentrations of both the hormone and its active metabolites, but current

---

TABLE 3.2

Causes of hypogonadism

Hypogonadotrophic (hypothalamic–pituitary dysfunction)

- Drugs, e.g. luteinizing hormone-releasing hormone analogues
- Pituitary tumour
- Congenital – Kallmann's syndrome
- Prader-Willi syndrome
- Bilateral orchidectomy

Hypergonadotrophic (primary testicular failure)

- Gonadal dysgenesis
- Rudimentary testis syndrome
- Congenital – Klinefelter's syndrome

androgen replacement therapies do not always achieve this.

In addition, androgen replacement therapy carries a potential risk of stimulating prostate growth and promoting the development of latent foci of prostate cancer. Although it is difficult to quantify these risks, and they are probably small, it is important that any patient receiving this treatment should be fully informed, and his PSA level monitored.

Vacuum devices and surgical options. These two treatment options are covered in detail on pages 47–9 and 50–7, respectively.

CHAPTER 4

Pharmacological treatment

Greater understanding of the physiological mechanism of erection and the role of smooth muscle relaxation led to the concept of the pharmacologically induced erection as a form of treatment for ED. During the early 1980s, it was established that drugs that relax cavernosal smooth muscle and/or reduce adrenergic sympathetic tone to the penile vasculature induce an erection if administered locally in adequate concentrations. The effects of papaverine, which is a powerful smooth muscle relaxant, were discovered after accidental intracavernous injection during a surgical procedure. Similar physiological and clinical observations led to a number of drugs being studied as potential therapeutic agents for ED (Table 4.1).

TABLE 4.1

Drugs with therapeutic potential in ED

Mechanism of action	Drug
Smooth muscle relaxation	Papaverine
	Nitroglycerine
	Verapamil
	Vasoactive intestinal polypeptide
	Alprostadil
α-adrenoceptor blockade	Phentolamine
	Phenoxybenzamine
	Yohimbine
	Moxisylyte
Phosphodiesterase type 5 inhibition	Sildenafil
Central nervous system activity	Apomorphine
	Trazodone

Oral pharmacological agents

Sildenafil citrate (Viagra®) is a breakthrough therapy in the treatment of ED. Nitric oxide, the key neurotransmitter involved in relaxation of corpus cavernosal smooth muscle, acts through a second messenger system involving guanylate cyclase. The cGMP produced is normally broken down by a cGMP-specific PDE 5 (see pages 11–14), which exists principally in the corpus cavernosa. Sildenafil is a selective inhibitor of PDE 5 and therefore enhances the normal vasodilatory erectile mechanisms (Figure 4.1).

Sildenafil has been evaluated in controlled clinical trials involving more than 3000 men aged 19–87 years. The mean duration of ED in these men was 5 years and aetiologies were organic, psychogenic or mixed. The agent works in response to natural sexual stimulation to improve erectile function. Treatment-related improvements in erections were reported by 70–90% of patients receiving sildenafil, versus 10–30% of men receiving placebo. Doses of 50 mg and 100 mg were well tolerated and highly effective in restoring erectile function in flexible-dose studies (Figure 4.2). Study results from more than 550 patients treated for at least 1 year indicate that the efficacy of sildenafil is maintained during long-term treatment (Figure 4.3).

Clinical trial data also demonstrate that sildenafil, taken 1 hour before sexual activity, is effective therapy for ED in a wide variety of patients,

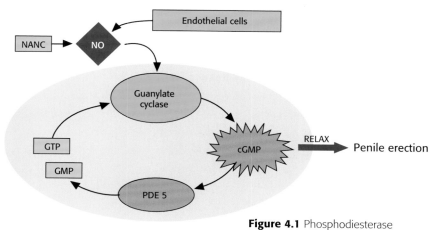

NO   Nitric oxide
NANC   Nonadrenergic–noncholinergic neurones
GTP   Guanosine triphosphate

Figure 4.1 Phosphodiesterase type 5 inhibition prevents cGMP breakdown and thereby enhances the normal erectile response.

35

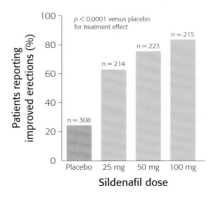

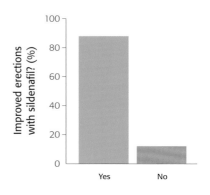

Figure 4.2 Patients treated with sildenafil reported improved erections in clinical trials.

Figure 4.3 After 1 year, most patients still reported improved erections with sildenafil.

including those with diabetes (57%), spinal cord injury (80%), as well as other concomitant medical disorders, such as hypertension (70%). It is also effective in patients taking a wide variety of other medications.

The recommended dose of sildenafil is 50 mg taken approximately 60 minutes before sexual activity; this should be taken no more than once daily. Based on efficacy and tolerance, the dose may be increased to 100 mg or reduced to 25 mg.

Side-effects and interactions. The adverse events reported in clinical trials with sildenafil were usually transient and mild to moderate in nature. The most commonly reported side-effects were mild and transient headache, flushing, dyspepsia and nasal congestion. Altered vision, such as temporary and subtle change in colour or brightness perception, was also reported in a small number of patients; this effect is thought to be due to some inhibitory effect of sildenafil on phosphodiesterase type 6, which is present in the photosensory cells of the retina. No cases of priapism were reported in these studies. The overall discontinuation from sildenafil therapy was low – 2.5% compared with 2.3% for those receiving placebo.

Sildenafil is cleared predominantly by cytochrome p450 isozymes in the liver. Cytochrome p450 inhibitors, such as cimetidine, ketoconazole and erythromycin, result in reduced clearance of sildenafil, but this is not usually associated with an increase in adverse events in patients taking this type of medication.

Sildenafil has peripheral vasodilatory properties, resulting in modest decreases in blood pressure in some patients. Consistent with its known effects on the nitric oxide/cGMP pathway, sildenafil is contraindicated in patients using nitrates, such as glyceryl trinitrate and isosorbide, or nitric oxide donors, such as sodium nitroprusside, in any form.

Yohimbine is derived from the bark of the *Pausinystalin yohimbe* tree which, for over a century, has been thought to possess aphrodisiac qualities. Yohimbine has well-defined properties as an α_2-adrenoceptor blocking agent, acting both peripherally and centrally. In a small study of men with psychogenic impotence, yohimbine has produced a positive response rate of 31% compared with only 5% with placebo; however, in a controlled trial in patients with organic ED, it was found to be no more effective than placebo.

This success has stimulated research into other α_2-blockers with the potential to produce a better response, and drugs with other actions.

Phentolamine is an α-adrenoceptor antagonist that has been used successfully in combination with other agents for intracorporal injection. Experience of its use as buccal preparation taken 15 minutes prior to intercourse suggested that adequate serum levels for a therapeutic response could be achieved through the oral route of administration. There is now an oral form of phentolamine, taken in doses between 40 and 80 mg, which has undergone placebo-controlled trials. The drug has a dose–response effect in men with ED from all aetiologies, with over 30% achieving an erection lasting until ejaculation. Side-effects are very similar to those found for yohimbine and other α-blockers, and include tachycardia, hypotension and headache.

Apomorphine is a dopamine-receptor agonist and acts on the dopaminergic receptors of the paraventricular nucleus of the hypothalamus. A sublingual form of apomorphine has been developed and is currently undergoing Phase III studies; early evidence suggests that it is an effective drug for men with psychogenic ED. In a recent placebo-controlled study, efficacy was demonstrated for men with mainly psychogenic ED. A dose–response effect was apparent between 2 and 6 mg, though side-effects were more common at the higher doses. At 6 mg, 21% of men needed to take a regular anti-emetic. The drug stimulates post-synaptic dopamine receptors in the hypothalamus, and thus needs to be taken on a regular basis.

Trazodone. The observation that certain patients developed priapism after taking the antidepressant trazodone led to its evaluation as a treatment for ED. A number of studies have suggested erectogenic activity in men with organic and psychogenic ED, though few have clearly shown statistically significant advantage over placebo. It may act as a serotonin-receptor antagonist, though it is also known to have some α-adrenoceptor antagonist activity. Side-effects include drowsiness and nausea.

Vasoactive drug therapy

Intracavernosal and intraurethral vasoactive drug therapy is particularly effective in men with any form of neurogenic dysfunction. These men have a normal haemodynamic mechanism, but lack the control system that initiates the erectile response; this can, however, be stimulated by any of the vasoactive agents. This observation is true for any of the neurogenic causes of ED including diabetic autonomic neuropathy. Psychogenic ED, which can also be regarded as a failure of appropriate neurotransmission to the erectile tissues, will often also respond very favourably to this treatment.

As experience with these agents has increased, men with other causes of ED have been treated, in particular men with vascular insufficiency who form the largest organic aetiological group in an ED clinic. High local concentrations of smooth muscle relaxant drugs act on both the trabecular muscle and the arteriolar vasculature and are able to overcome mild arterial insufficiency. However, when the arterial supply is severely compromised, pharmacologically induced arterial dilatation is ineffective because it cannot facilitate sufficient inflow to engorge the lacunar spaces and operate the veno-occlusive mechanism.

Although all vasoactive drugs produce some degree of erectile response when injected directly into the corpus cavernosum, so far only five have found widespread clinical use: papaverine, phentolamine, prostaglandin E_1, moxisylyte and VIP. The others have failed to do so due to either lack of efficacy or side-effects caused by leakage of the drug into the systemic circulation.

Intracavernosal therapy

The efficacy and safety of self-injection with vasoactive drugs has been demonstrated by the dramatic increase in their use over the last 10 years; the overall use of intracorporal self-injection continues to increase and alprostadil has now been approved by many regulatory authorities. Originally used only by patients with neurogenic impairment, such as spinal cord injuries, this form of treatment has since proved to be effective for men with many other types of erectile disorder (Table 4.2).

Papaverine is a powerful direct smooth muscle relaxant that acts on both the trabecular muscle of the erectile tissue and the vascular tone, inducing an erection that lasts for several hours. Since the introduction of vasoactive agents, papaverine has been the most widely used agent for intracorporal self-injection. It has been extensively studied and shown to be effective. Data from over 4000 men in clinical trials have shown that about 70% of all men who attended an ED clinic obtained an erection sufficient for sexual intercourse. The dose necessary to achieve this can vary from 10 mg to 80 mg, and it is necessary to titrate the dose up to an effective level for each patient to avoid the risk of priapism. For those men who have failed to get an adequate response from papaverine alone, combination therapy with phentolamine and papaverine may prove beneficial. Phentolamine, acting directly on the α-adrenoceptors of the vascular smooth muscle, potentiates the effects of papaverine.

Phentolamine acts principally to reduce adrenergically induced vascular smooth muscle tone, and probably does not initiate an erection on its own.

TABLE 4.2

Indications for intracorporal self-injection with vasoactive drugs

Good response

- Psychogenic ED
- Diabetes mellitus
- Neurogenic ED

Moderate response

- Mild arterial insufficiency
- Drug-induced ED
- Mild veno-occlusive disorder
- Age-related ED

Poor response

- Severe arterial insufficiency
- Very elderly men
- Severe veno-occlusive disorder

It is used in combination with papaverine and appears to work synergistically with it.

Prostaglandin E$_1$. In 1913, it was established that an extract of human prostate, called prostaglandin, was able to reduce blood pressure. By 1985, prostaglandin E$_1$ was isolated (alprostadil) and had been shown to cause relaxation of smooth muscle in the corpus cavernosum via an adenylate cyclase second messenger system. It is a natural body constituent found in high concentrations in the seminal vesicles and corpora cavernosa, and is actively metabolized in the lung (70% first-pass metabolism), liver and kidney. Alprostadil acts by inhibiting α-adrenergic tone in the penile vasculature and by relaxing trabecular smooth muscle.

Recently, alprostadil has become the drug of choice for intracavernous pharmacotherapy. Prostaglandin E$_1$ plays a role as a neurotransmitter in the natural erectile mechanism, and alprostadil is at least as effective in treating ED as combination therapy with papaverine and phentolamine, and appears to have fewer side-effects. As a result, the alprostadil preparations Caverject® and Viridal Duo® have been licensed for the treatment of ED in Europe and the USA. There are now data on over 10,000 men with ED who have undergone self-injection with alprostadil. In one study of 550 men, over 70% of patients achieved an erection sufficient for sexual intercourse that lasted for at least 30 minutes and, in another study, 77% of sexual partners reported the erections to be 'good' or 'very good', with 74% reporting an improvement in their relationship. Once again the final therapeutic dose of drug must be titrated up to prevent the risk of priapism, although this risk is considerably less than that with papaverine. The effective dose can range from 5 μg to 20 μg depending on the aetiology of the ED. Occasionally, larger doses (up to 60 μg) are required.

Moxisylyte is an α$_1$-blocker that acts on the normal sympathetic tone to maintain penile flaccidity. This treatment option is indicated in men with raised sympathetic tone associated with internal stress and anxiety. Published results suggest that although it appears to have an overall lower efficacy than other injectable agents (46% of patients achieving success in the home), it also has a lower local side-effect profile and is thus well tolerated by patients. Patients with psychogenic causes seem to respond best, though they may require the higher dose of drug (20 mg) to overcome the sympathetic tone. The incidence of side-effects at this higher dose are not increased, with local pain on injection being rare and prolonged erections affecting less than 1%.

Vasoactive intestinal polypeptide is a neurotransmitter that acts on the adenylate cyclase system of the smooth muscle cell, reducing intracellular calcium and initiating relaxation. When used in isolation as an intracavernosal agent, it has a lower efficacy than other injectable agents but has been shown to be very effective in combination with phentolamine. In a study of over 550 men with predominantly organic ED, 83% were able to achieve erections with one of the two doses available. Adverse events were uncommon, with prolonged erections occurring in only 3 men, and pain on injection was rarely reported. Phentolamine–VIP and the injector device are well tolerated by patients and partners alike. The combination has undergone Phase III trials and is awaiting regulatory approval at the time of press.

Combination therapy. In men who fail to get an adequate response from papaverine alone, combination therapy with phentolamine, papaverine and prostaglandin E_1 often proves beneficial. Phentolamine, acting directly on the α-adrenoceptors of the vascular smooth muscle, appears to potentiate the effects of papaverine.

Other vasoactive drugs and drug combinations, such as the combination of phentolamine and VIP, are being introduced and their therapeutic potential is currently under evaluation. The vasoactive agents discussed here can also be used in combination with sildenafil.

Contraindications. Papaverine, phentolamine and alprostadil have a low rate of leakage into the systemic circulation, resulting in few contraindications to their use. There are, however, some relative contraindications (Table 4.3).

Self-injection technique. Many patients attending an ED clinic will be given a trial injection of a vasoactive drug in an effort not only to establish the possible origin of their problem, but also to test the efficacy of the drug as a potential therapy. If efficacy is proven and the patient wishes to proceed, then he will need to be taught the self-injection technique (Figure 4.4).

TABLE 4.3

Relative contraindications to vasoactive drug therapy

- Sickle cell trait or disease
- Leukaemia
- Anticoagulation
- Poor manual dexterity
- Blood-borne infections, such as HIV or hepatitis
- Previous history of priapism

The person who demonstrates the technique should administer increasing doses of the vasoactive agent of choice until a good quality erection is obtained. With alprostadil, the recommended starting dose is 1.25 µg for patients with known neurogenic or psychogenic impotence, and 2.5 µg for others, with the dose being doubled on each successive injection. With papaverine, the starting point may be 5 mg, increasing in 5 mg increments.

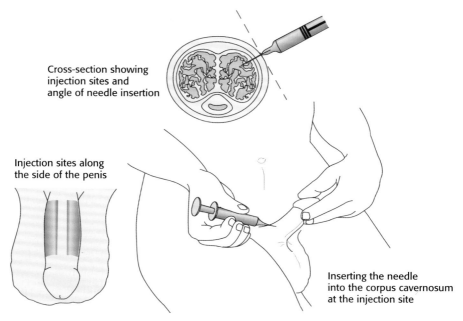

Cross-section showing injection sites and angle of needle insertion

Injection sites along the side of the penis

Inserting the needle into the corpus cavernosum at the injection site

Figure 4.4 Self-injection technique.

These recommendations are suitable for patients with suspected neurogenic or psychogenic ED, but if there is known arterial insufficiency, the starting dose is usually higher. When a satisfactory erection is achieved, the patient and his partner will gain confidence with the technique.

First, the patient, or his partner, must become familiar with the handling of the needles and syringes and the technique of drawing up drug solutions. In addition, alprostadil needs to be reconstituted from powder prior to injection. The skin over the penis is drawn taut, and the needle and syringe held at right angles to the penis (Figure 4.4). The injection is given near to the base of the penis on either side and avoiding any visible veins. Injection sites should be varied. Teaching demonstrations, illustrated manuals and videos, which are all available from the manufacturers, are recommended.

Side-effects from self-injection of vasoactive agents (Table 4.4) can be classified as:
- treatment failure
- unwanted local effects
- unwanted vasodilatory systemic effects (e.g. flushing and hypotension).

Treatment failure. The most common side-effect is treatment failure: 80% of failures are due to incorrect administration of the drug into the corpora cavernosa, usually as a result of incorrect injection technique. If injections continue to be ineffective despite correct technique, a higher drug dose may be necessary. Systemic side-effects are uncommon (about 1%) and result from leakage of the drug into the circulation. Phentolamine has been reported to occasionally cause dizziness, tachycardia and hypotension, as has alprostadil, and papaverine has been associated with occasional

TABLE 4.4

Comparison of side-effects of injectable agents

	Moxisylyte (%)	Alprostadil (%)	VIP plus phentolamine (%)
Priapism	< 0.5	0.5 – 1.3	< 0.5
Pain on injection	10	17 – 50	1
Haematoma	3	3	3
Systemic effects	2	1	10 – 50

derangement of liver function. These observations have not led to any significant limitation in the use of these agents.

Priapism. The most troublesome side-effect with any of these drugs is the development of a prolonged erection, or priapism. Any erection lasting for 4 hours or more, especially if painful, should be regarded as a priapism and treatment should be sought. Patients *must* be pre-warned of this potential complication, both verbally and in writing, and should be given instructions on what they should do in the event of a priapism. The occurrence of priapism is dose-dependent with each of the drugs, and tends to occur during the early stages of titration during a treatment programme. Published data indicate that priapism is more common with papaverine, or a combination of papaverine and phentolamine, than with alprostadil. The incidence of priapism after injection with alprostadil has been reported to be between 0.5% and 1.3%, but is between 2.3% and 15% after papaverine.

If a priapism does occur, medical intervention should be sought within 6–8 hours. Failure to achieve detumescence after 6–8 hours can cause irreversible ischaemic damage to the corpora cavernosa with subsequent fibrotic damage and permanent loss of erectile function. In most cases, priapism can be relieved by simple aspiration of blood (in 50–100 ml portions) through an appropriate calibre needle placed in the corpora cavernosa. If the priapism persists, injection of a dilute solution of an α-agonist, such as phenylephrine or metaraminol, into the corpora cavernosa should be tried, though the patient's heart rate and blood pressure should be carefully monitored because of the risk of tachycardia and hypertension. Surgical intervention is required only if the priapism is particularly prolonged (i.e. > 12 hours); surgery involves the creation of a vascular shunt between the corpora cavernosa and the systemic circulation, usually the corpus spongiosum, and is itself associated with subsequent ED.

Other local side-effects. Include the formation of fibrotic nodules around the injection site after repeated use (which can lead to penile curvature), haematoma formation, and the presence of diffuse pain along the shaft of the penis immediately after injection. Discomfort in the penile shaft is thought to be more common with the use of alprostadil than the other vasoactive drugs, but this does not often result in the cessation of therapy.

Intraurethral therapy

Alprostadil has been developed for insertion into the urethra as a pellet through a specific polypropylene applicator. Once delivered, the pellet dissolves into the urethral mucosa.

Alprostadil is a synthetic form of prostaglandin E_1; it acts via the adenylate cyclase system to reduce intracellular calcium and induce smooth muscle relaxation. The system for this administration of alprostadil is marketed as MUSE® (Medicated Urethral System for Erection; Figure 4.5). Before use, men are asked to urinate as this aids insertion of the applicator and facilitates dispersion of the drug. While in the sitting position, the patient inserts the applicator and then depresses the ejector button, releasing the alprostadil pellet. The penis is then held upright and gently rolled to disperse the drug. Erections develop about 10–15 minutes after application and last for approximately 30 minutes.

Early results with this treatment show a dose–response effect, with 66% of men with ED (all causes) obtaining a full erection, though subsequent studies have reported a lower efficacy. The doses required to achieve this ranged from 125 to 1000 µg. The side-effects of this treatment are those of urethral pain (7%) and minor urethral trauma (1%). In a comparative study of intracavernosal and intraurethral application of alprostadil, the intracavernosal administration was shown to be more effective though there was a slightly higher incidence of local side-effects than with the intraurethral route of administration. It would thus seem that while the intraurethral route of administration is associated with a lower overall success rate, the improved side-effect profile and acceptability to patients may make it a preferred option for some patients.

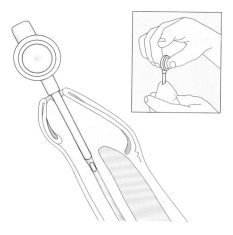

Figure 4.5 Intraurethral administration of alprostadil using the MUSE® system.

Androgen replacement therapy for hypogonadal men

Oral administration. Two types of oral testosterone are available – modified and unmodified. Unmodified testosterone is rapidly absorbed and degraded by the liver, making it difficult to achieve satisfactory serum concentrations. Modified 17-alkyltestosterones, such as methyltestosterone or fluoxymesterone, usually require large doses and multiple daily dose regimens. In addition, these compounds are associated with idiosyncratic hepatotoxicity, even at relatively low doses.

Intramuscular injection. Testosterone is esterified for intramuscular administration to prevent rapid degradation and to render it more soluble in oily vehicles (which carry the drug in muscle tissue). Although until recently intramuscular administration was the delivery method of choice, there are a number of significant drawbacks. These include abnormally high initial serum concentrations of testosterone and oestradiol, followed by a decline to subnormal levels before the next injection. Testosterone depot therapy has been reported to produce positive and negative fluctuations in libido, erectile function, energy and mood, in parallel with the variations in serum androgen levels. In addition, patients often find deep intramuscular injections painful and dislike the frequent visits to the surgery that are required.

Testosterone skin patches. Several forms of testosterone skin patch are now approved. Controlled transdermal delivery has been used effectively to provide hormone replacement therapy in women, smoking cessation therapy and to treat angina. In hypogonadal men, daily application of testosterone patches produces hormone levels that parallel the endogenous pattern of serum testosterone characteristic of normal men. Patients report improvements in mood, energy, libido and sexual function to a statistically significant greater extent than seen with placebo. The only side-effects are transient local itching, skin irritation and discomfort related to the patch.

CHAPTER 5

Vacuum devices

The vacuum constriction device is one of the most time-honoured methods of treating ED. Its design was first patented in 1917 by Dr Otto Lederer and, although the construction and design of the devices has become more sophisticated, the concept remains the same – a vacuum is applied to the penis for a few minutes, causing tumescence and rigidity, which is sustained using a constricting ring at the base of the penis.

Physiology

The physiological changes that occur in a penis during a vacuum-induced erection are quite different from those that occur during a normal or even a pharmacologically induced erection. Trabecular smooth muscle relaxation does not occur; blood is simply trapped in both the intracorporal and extracorporal compartments of the penis. Distal to the constricting band of the device, venous stasis and decreased arterial inflow lead to penile distension, but also to cyanosis, oedema and a progressive drop in skin temperature. Consequently, vacuum-induced erections eventually become uncomfortable and should not be maintained for more than 30 minutes. In addition, the penis only becomes rigid distal to the constricting bands, rather than along the whole corporal length. As a result, the penis tends to pivot inconveniently at its base.

Equipment and technique

Although many different devices are now manufactured, they all have three common components: a vacuum chamber, a pump and a constriction band that is applied to the base of the penis once an erection is achieved (Figure 5.1). The vacuum chamber is made of clear plastic and is open at one end. This is placed over the penis and, with the help of a lubricant jelly, a seal is formed between the chamber and skin, and the pump mechanism then creates a vacuum of at least 100 mmHg, which draws in sufficient blood to create an erection (Figure 5.2). The pump mechanism may be either attached to the vacuum chamber itself or separate from it, and may be either hand or battery operated. Once an erection develops, an elastic ring (the constriction

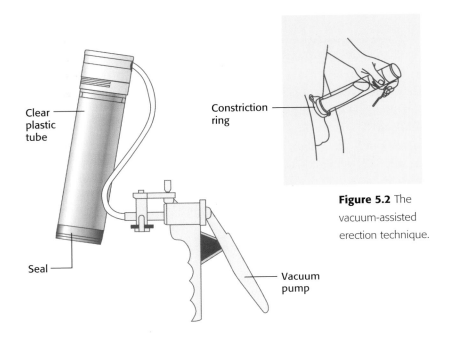

Clear plastic tube

Seal

Constriction ring

Figure 5.2 The vacuum-assisted erection technique.

Vacuum pump

Figure 5.1 A typical vacuum erection device which is placed over the penis and used to induce an erection that is maintained with a constriction ring.

band) slips off the chamber and maintains the rigidity by preventing blood escape without injury to the penis. These constriction rings are available in a variety of different sizes.

Clinical use

Because the mechanism of erection is non-physiological, the vacuum constriction device is theoretically suitable for most men who experience ED. Indeed, in one study, 98% of men were able to achieve an erection sufficient for sexual intercourse using one of these devices. In clinical practice, the proportion of men who successfully use this technique is about the same as that who find satisfaction with intracavernosal self-injection. In one report, men who responded well to papaverine were the same group of men who responded well to the vacuum device. As with self-injection, there are some instances when caution should be observed (Table 5.1).

TABLE 5.1

Relative contraindications to the use of vacuum devices

- Sickle cell trait or disease
- Leukaemia
- Anticoagulation, bleeding disorders
- Poor manual dexterity

Side-effects

Complications arising from the use of these devices are generally of a minor nature. Petechiae due to capillary rupture are common and transient (10%); haematoma formation is less common (about 5% of patients) and often associated with application of a vacuum pressure that is too high. Other complaints from men using these devices include numbness in the penis (occurring in 75% of users at some stage), a feeling of cold, blue discoloration of the penis and altered or diminished sensation of orgasm (Table 5.2). Orgasm is often dry, due to the constriction ring which compresses the urethra and so prevents normal ejaculation and often causes some discomfort. Users have also commented on the lack of spontaneity of sexual relations associated with the use of these devices. Despite these complaints, men do not seem to be deterred from using vacuum devices and most studies show a reasonable rate of patient and partner satisfaction (68–83%) with the technique.

TABLE 5.2

Side-effects of vacuum devices

Numbness/penis feels cold	75%
Lack of ejaculation	50%
Altered sensation at orgasm	25%
Haematoma/petechiae formation	15%
Discomfort on orgasm	9–11%

CHAPTER 6

Surgical treatment

Surgical treatment of ED is usually reserved for patients in whom more conservative therapy has failed, or for whom conservative therapy is contraindicated. Most of these patients will have significant arterial or venous disease, penile corpus cavernosum fibrosis, or will, by choice, prefer the prospect of a 'one-off' solution. Three surgical options are available:

• implantation of a penile prosthesis
• ligation for venous incompetence
• vascular bypass surgery for arterial or venous abnormalities.

While the outcome of surgical intervention may be more reliable in certain selected patients, the incidence of morbidity and complications is significantly greater than with medical treatment.

Penile prosthetic implants

Surgically implantable penile prostheses are classified as either semi-rigid or inflatable. Many types with various modifications are widely available. Implants provide penile rigidity and erectile size that adequately simulate the normal physiological erectile state required for sexual intercourse. After careful assessment and discussion with the patient and his partner on their preference, the implants are sized during surgery. The degree of flaccidity differs according to the type of device selected.

Semi-rigid rod prostheses

Semi-rigid rod devices were the first prostheses designed to restore erections and erectile function, and are still used extensively. A variety of semi-rigid rod penile prostheses of different designs are currently available. These prostheses consist of two flexible rods or cylinders that can be varied in length by trimming the proximal portion or adding measured extensions to the proximal portion to fit the individual patient's measurements (Figure 6.1). Curvature is adjusted via the flexibility provided in their design which usually includes a central, braided metal wire allowing upward or downward deviation of the prosthesis. Mechanical modifications of these devices include hinges to increase the flexibility and ability to position the prosthesis.

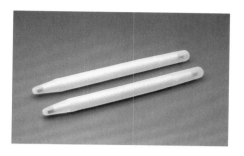

Figure 6.1 Semi-rigid rod penile prostheses are implanted into the corpora cavernosa. They comprise two rods that are trimmed in length intra-operatively, fitted in width, and adjusted in curvature through the flexibility provided in their design.

Surgical implantation of these semi-rigid rod prostheses is the simplest type of procedure. A dorsal, subcoronal penile incision, a penoscrotal incision (Figure 6.2), ventral penile incision, or a perineal incision may be used to access the corpora cavernosa for dilatation of the corpora and implantation.

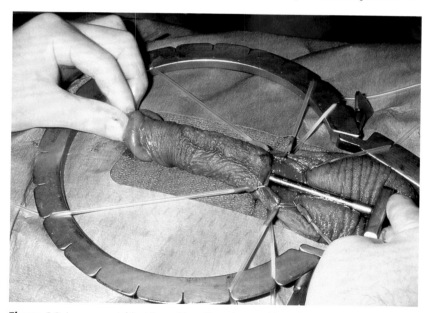

Figure 6.2 A penoscrotal incision with a dilator inserted into the right corpus cavernosum to create the space needed to insert a penile prosthesis.

Inflatable penile prostheses

Inflatable penile prostheses are available in self-contained, two-piece, and three-piece designs (Figures 6.3–6.5).

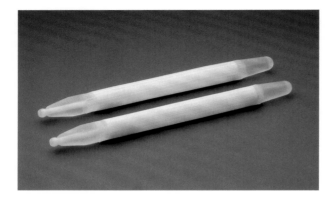

Figure 6.3
Self-contained inflatable prostheses with a pump on the distal tip of each cylinder.

Figure 6.4
A two-piece inflatable prosthesis with a combined pump and reservoir.

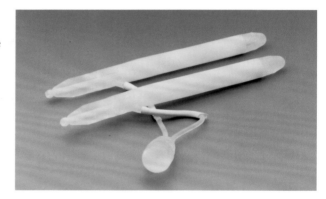

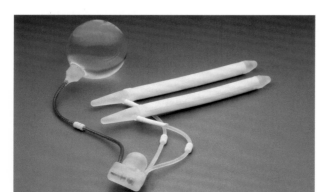

Figure 6.5
A three-piece inflatable implant showing the separate pump, reservoir and cylinders.

Self-contained inflatable penile prostheses are modifications of semi-rigid and inflatable prostheses in which each cylinder contains an inflation chamber, pump and proximal reservoir. The device is inflated by pressure on the distal portion of each cylinder just proximal to the glans penis. This pressure fills each cylinder with saline supplied from the proximal reservoir. Although little distension of these cylinders occurs, rigidity can be expected from appropriate inflation. Deflation is achieved by exerting external pressure on the cylinders by deflecting them downwards. A release valve in the pump mechanism allows fluid to return from the inflatable portion of the prosthesis to the reservoir as the pressure is increased, thereby deflating the device. These prostheses are implanted in the same way as semi-rigid rod prostheses.

Two-piece inflatable penile prostheses contain two completely inflatable cylinders and a pump/reservoir. This pump/reservoir provides a limited, but usually adequate, volume of fluid for inflation and deflation of the prosthesis. The two-piece design avoids the need for an abdominal fluid reservoir, which is used in three-piece inflatable prostheses. The two-piece design also has an advantage over the self-contained prostheses by increasing the volume of fluid placed in the penile cylinders to improve both erectile inflation and flaccidity. Because of the size of the pump/reservoir, however, flaccidity may not be as complete as with the three-piece inflatable prostheses. Implantation of this device is similar to that described below for the three-piece inflatable penile prosthesis.

Three-piece inflatable penile prostheses are the most complex, yet most cosmetic penile prosthetic devices available. Two inflatable cylinders are placed in the hollow corpora cavernosa and connected to a small pump device placed in the scrotum lateral to the testicle, which is used to inflate and deflate the cylinders, thereby simulating a normal erection (Figures 6.6 and 6.7). Saline is provided from a reservoir placed beneath the rectus muscles of the abdomen. Because of the significant volume provided by this reservoir for both inflation and deflation, both the erect and flaccid states produced are usually excellent. The three-piece inflatable prosthesis provides increased girth and length in comparison to other devices and the more natural flaccid state facilitates the positioning and carriage of the prosthesis under clothing.

53

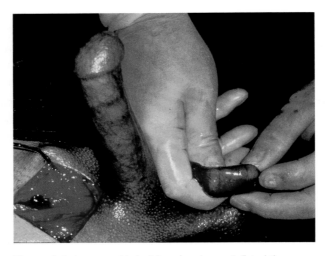

Figure 6.6 A suprapubic incision showing an inflated three-piece prosthesis.

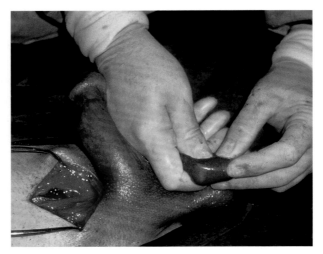

Figure 6.7 A three-piece prosthesis being deflated.

Postoperative care

An ice pack is applied to the genitalia after the operation, and patients are treated with antibiotics to prevent infection. Oral analgesics are also administered. In addition, with inflatable devices, patients are asked to check the position of the pump for 4–6 weeks before activation to maintain its dependent position in the scrotum. Patients are then asked to return to learn how to activate and deflate the device 6 weeks after the operation.

Postoperative complications. Although the incidence of postoperative complications has decreased markedly over the past decade, mechanical malfunction can still occur with any of the penile prosthetic devices. The semi-rigid rod penile prostheses may require replacement due to cable fracture, or reduced rigidity. Inflatable prostheses are, however, more likely to suffer mechanical complications, although reported mechanical malfunction rates are currently less than 5% over 3 years. Fluid leakage is the most common problem with inflatable prostheses; fluid leaks most commonly occur in the cylinders, which are the portion of the device under the highest pressure. In all cases, device malfunction requires surgical exploration and replacement of the faulty parts of the prosthesis.

Another potential complication is infection; this occurs in 3–5% of patients with penile prostheses. Higher infection rates can be expected in patients who have had alterations or repairs to their prosthesis, and those with autoimmune diseases and diabetes mellitus. Prosthesis removal, healing, and subsequent replacement is the usual procedure for patients with infection. Other complications that can arise include erosion of the prosthesis, sustained pain, reduced penile length and reduction in sensation. These complications, though rare, are of significant concern to those men affected and their partners, as well as the surgeon involved.

Patient and partner satisfaction

A number of studies have assessed the outcome and the degree of postoperative satisfaction of patients undergoing penile prosthesis implantation. In general, satisfaction rates are high with all types of implant. The success of surgical treatment is linked to expectations as well as the relationship between the patient and his partner, and the psychological state of the patient preoperatively. One study comparing satisfaction rates identified no significant difference in patient satisfaction with the semi-rigid and inflatable devices, but when the patients' sexual partners were included in the survey, increased satisfaction with inflatable implants was noted.

Surgery for venous incompetence

Surgical procedures for venous incompetence are designed to increase venous outflow resistance in the sinusoidal spaces of the corpora cavernosa. Prior to these surgical procedures, patients are evaluated using cavernosography and cavernosometry, in which contrast medium is infused continuously into the corpora cavernosa. The use of these diagnostic tests after injection with a vasoactive agent will confirm that the patient's ED is due to venous leakage or incompetence. Patients with veno-occlusive dysfunction typically complain of firm erections for short periods of time (which they describe as partial and fleeting).

Such patients may be candidates for surgery to correct venous incompetence if studies of arterial inflow demonstrate normal arterial function; surgical treatment may involve crural plication, deep penile dorsal vein excision and ligation, or dorsal vein arterialization.

The outcomes of surgical intervention to correct ED caused by venous incompetence have been poor. Surgical success has been achieved in less than 40% of patients with an additional 40% responding to a combination of surgery and injectable vasoactive agents. Postoperative complications include penile shortening, decreased penile sensation, recurrent venous incompetence and wound infection. Due to the very variable success of these procedures, venous ligation procedures should be performed only in carefully selected patients who are fully informed of the limited success rate and the risk of complications.

Arterial revascularization

As high blood flow rates produce erectile function in the corpora cavernosa, the integrity of the arterial supply is critical for normal erectile function. Patients with arterial lesions (usually acquired traumatically) in whom there is no significant atherosclerosis or atherosclerotic risk factors may therefore be suitable for penile arterial revascularization or deep dorsal vein arterialization. Specific arteriographic visualization of the internal pudendal arteries and central cavernosal arteries is, however, essential to diagnose arterial compromise. Once diagnostic studies have demonstrated arterial abnormalities, arteriography following stimulation of the corpus cavernosum with vasoactive agents will document arterial abnormalities in the internal iliac vessels. Arterial revascularization should also be considered in lesions unlikely to respond to percutaneous transluminal angioplasty.

The alternative forms of surgical intervention must be discussed with all patients selected for arterial revascularization, including the possibility of penile prosthesis implantation.

Arterial revascularization can be achieved using a variety of procedures, each of which depends on the use of the inferior epigastric artery. As the central cavernosal arteries are relatively inaccessible for revascularization, one of the dorsal arteries is a better choice for anastomosis with the inferior epigastric artery. This can be performed in an end-to-end or end-to-side fashion with distal ligation of the dorsal artery of the penis to redirect blood to central cavernosal arteries.

Although this procedure usually has few complications, excessive arterial blood flow may result in priapism or glans penis hyperaemia, and the anastomosis may occlude during the postoperative period. Patients are encouraged to avoid sexual activity for approximately 6 weeks after the operation.

The results of these procedures vary widely, but up to 65% of patients have reported a return of erectile function following arterial bypass grafts although this is not always sustained. With careful selection of patients, good surgical technique, and long-term follow up, outcomes may improve.

CHAPTER 7

Associated medical conditions

A number of medical conditions are commonly associated with ED, including:
- diabetes mellitus
- hypertension
- vascular disease
- endocrine abnormalities.

Other situations and conditions are associated with ED, though the link is not recognized. Awareness of them should mean patients can be warned of the risk of ED, and early diagnosis and treatment can occur.

Peyronie's disease

Peyronie's disease is curvature of the penis due to fibrosis within the tunica albuginea. The affected corpora cavernosa cannot lengthen on erection, leading to curvature. The condition is most common in middle-aged men who are sexually active. Its exact aetiology remains unknown, but it may result from trauma and bleeding into the tunica, followed by activation of the inflammatory process and fibrosis. The more recent observation that HLA class II antigens are more common in men with Peyronie's disease suggests an underlying autoimmune cause. Erectile dysfunction occurs in 30–40% of men with Peyronie's disease. Although the mechanism of their ED is not clearly understood, most appear to have a vascular problem, such as arterial insufficiency where the fibrosis actually distorts the vessels, or failure of the veno-occlusive mechanism.

To a certain extent, treatment is determined by whether the patient has ED and Peyronie's disease. If the patient has this combination, he is probably best advised to undergo insertion of a penile implant, as surgical straightening of the penis alone is unlikely to overcome the ED. If penile curvature alone is the factor that precludes intercourse, surgical correction of the curvature by plaque excision and grafting, or the Nesbit operation is favoured. This latter procedure involves shortening of the contralateral corpus cavernosum. Patients should be warned of the risks of penile shortening and onset of ED after surgery.

Renal failure

Chronic renal impairment is associated with a high incidence of ED, with the incidence increasing with the level of creatinine. Erectile dysfunction is present in about 50% of patients by the time they require dialysis. A number of factors may be involved, including:

- anaemia
- autonomic neuropathy
- reduced testosterone levels with elevated prolactin
- accelerated arterial disease
- other drug therapies
- psychological stress.

After successful transplantation and normalization of renal function, erectile function is restored in many patients. Erythropoietin treatment in patients with renal impairment can also improve the patient's overall quality of life and erectile function.

Pelvic surgery

Any form of pelvic surgery can lead to nerve damage affecting the erectile mechanism. The cavernous nerves run from the pelvic plexus on the lateral border of the rectum down behind the prostate and into the base of the penis. Damage is, therefore, most likely to occur following surgery to the rectum, bladder or prostate. Improved knowledge of the anatomical course of these nerves has led to the development of surgical techniques that aim to preserve them where possible, but damage cannot be avoided during some operations for malignant disease.

Patients who undergo gastrointestinal surgery that results in an ileostomy or colostomy may suffer depression or loss of self-esteem, which may cause ED. This is particularly relevant to sufferers of inflammatory bowel disease requiring excision of the rectum and ileostomy. Patients should always be made aware that specific surgical procedures may lead to ED (Table 7.1). Evidence suggests that the sooner pharmacological treatment is started after an operation, the more likely the patient is to regain normal erectile function.

Penile injuries

Damage to either the corpora cavernosa or to the neurovascular bundles that supply the corpora can lead to failure of the erectile mechanism. Recently, it has been suggested that cycling may cause traumatic injury to the pudendal nerves.

TABLE 7.1

Risks of ED associated with surgery

Procedure	Reported risks (%)
Radical prostatectomy	10–90
Radical cystectomy	50–90
TURP	8
Anterior resection of rectum	10–50

Corporal injuries

Blunt or penetrating injuries can cause rupture of the tunica albuginea. If not surgically repaired immediately, such injuries can lead to persistent venous leakage through the defect, causing failure of normal corporal filling. The most common cause of blunt trauma is penile fracture (i.e. rupture of the tunica albuginea). This occurs during sexual intercourse or masturbation, and is characterized by an audible crack, followed by penile pain, loss of erection and the onset of a penile haematoma.

Treatment involves urgent exploration and repair of the corporal defect, which should preserve potency in most cases. If repair is delayed for 36 hours or more, ED is a likely consequence.

Neurovascular bundle injuries

Urethral trauma is the most common cause of injury to the neurovascular bundle, after surgery. It may occur either after a perineal injury and bulbar urethral damage or a pelvic fracture injury and membranous urethral damage. In either instance, it is the neurovascular bundle running posterolateral to the apex of the prostate and posterior urethra that is disrupted. The further the injury is away from the membranous urethra, the less likely it is that ED will result. Thus anterior urethral trauma only occasionally results in this problem.

Complete urethral disruption injuries from a pelvic fracture are almost universally associated with ED, which may be difficult to treat. Patients often have a combination of both neurological and vascular impairment. Consequently, they do not often respond to conventional pharmacological treatments. In some cases, arterial revascularization surgery should be considered.

Key references

EPIDEMIOLOGY

Feldman HA, Goldstein I, Hatzichristou DG et al. Impotence and its medical and psychological correlates: results of the Massachusetts Male Aging Study. *J Urol* 1994;150:54–61.

Kinsey AC, Pomeroy W, Martin C. Age and sexual outlet. In: Kinsey AC, Pomeroy W, Martin C, eds. *Sexual behaviour in the human male.* Philadelphia: W. B. Saunders Co., 1948:218–262.

Lechtenderg R, Ohl DA. Effects of aging. In: Lechtenderg R, Ohl DA, eds. *Sexual Dysfunction.* Philadelphia: Lea and Febiger, 1994:183–188.

Maatman TJ, Montague DK, Martin LM. Erectile dysfunction in men with diabetes mellitus. *Urology* 1987;29:589–592.

NIH Consensus Development Panel on Impotence. *JAMA* 1993;270:83–90.

PATHOPHYSIOLOGY

Fournier GR, Juenemann KP, Lue TF, Tanagho EA. Mechanism of venous occlusion during canine penile erection. An anatomical demonstration. *J Urol* 1987;137:163–167.

Lerner SE, Melman A, Christ GJ. A review of erectile dysfunction: new insights and more questions. *J Urol* 1993;149: 1246–1255.

Lue TF, Tanagho EA. Functional anatomy and mechanism of penile erection. In: Lue TF, Tanagho EA, McClure RD, eds. *Contemporary management of impotence and infertility.* Baltimore: Williams and Wilkins, 1988:39–50.

Wagner G, Saenz de Tejeda I. Update on male erectile dysfunction. *Br Med J* 1998;316:678–82.

Walsh PC, Mostwin JL. Radical prostatectomy and cystoprostatectomy with preservation of potency: results using a new nerve-sparing technique. *Br J Urol* 1984;56:694–697.

DIAGNOSIS

Kirby RS. Impotence: diagnosis and management of erectile dysfunction. *BMJ* 1994;308:957–961.

Krane RJ. Medical progress. Impotence. *N Engl J Med* 1989;321:1648–1658.

Rosen RC, Riley A, Wagner G et al. The International Index of Erectile Function (IIEF): a multidimensional scale for the assessment of erectile dysfunction. *Urology* 1997;49:822–830.

PSYCHOGENIC ERECTILE DYSFUNCTION

Barnes P. Role of sex therapy in the management of erectile dysfunction. In: Kirby RS, Carson C, Webster GD, eds. *Impotence: diagnosis and management.* Oxford: Butterworth-Heinemann, 1991:133–142.

ORAL AGENTS

Boolell M, Gepi-Attee S, Gingell JC, Allen MJ. Sildenafil, a novel effective oral therapy for erectile dysfunction. *Br J Urol* 1996;78:257–261.

Eardley I. New oral therapies for the treatment of erectile dysfunction. *Br J Urol* 1998;81:122–127.

Goldstein I, Lue TF, Padma-Nathan H et al. Oral sildenafil in the treatment of erectile dysfunction. *N Eng J Med* 1998;338:1397–1404.

INTRACAVERNOSAL THERAPY

Eden CG, Bellringer JF, Carter PG et al. Managing impotence in diabetes. Two drugs are better than one. *BMJ* 1993;307:19–20.

Lee LM, Stevenson RW, Szasz G. Prostaglandin E1 versus phentolamine papaverine for the treatment of erectile impotence: a double-blind comparison. *J Urol* 1989;141:549–550.

Levine SB, Althof SE, Turner LA et al. Side-effects of self-administration of intracavernous papaverine and phentolamine for the treatment of impotence. *J Urol* 1989;141:54–57.

Linet OI, Ogring FG. Efficacy and safety of intracavernosal alprostadil in men with erectile dysfunction. *N Engl J Med* 1996;334:873–877.

Morales A, Heaton JP. The medical treatment of impotence: an update. *World J Urol* 1990;8:80–83.

Stakl W, Hasun R, Marberger M. Prostaglandin E1 in the treatment of erectile dysfunction. *World J Urol* 1990;8:84–86.

Virag R. Intracavernous injection of Papaverine for erectile failure. *Lancet* 1982;ii:938.

INTRAURETHRAL THERAPY

Padma-Nathan H, Hellstrom WJG, Kaiser FE et al. Treatment of men with erectile dysfunction with transurethral alprostadil. *N Engl J Med* 1997;336:1–7.

Padma-Nathan H et al. Multicenter, double-blind, placebo-controlled trial of transurethral alprostadil in men with chronic erectile dysfunction. *J Urol* 1996;155:Abstract 740.

Porst H. Transurethral alprostadil with MUSE vs intracavernous alprostadil – a comparative study in 103 patients with erectile dysfunction. *Int J Impot Res* 1997;9:187–192.

VACUUM DEVICES

Bodansky HJ. Treatment of erectile dysfunction using active vacuum assist devices. *Diabetic Med* 1994;11:410–412.

Bosshardt RJ, Farwerk R, Sikora R et al. Objective measurement of the effectiveness, therapeutic success and dynamic mechanisms of the vacuum device. *Br J Urol* 1995;75:786–791.

Nadig PW. Vacuum erection devices. A review. *World J Urol* 1990;8:114–117.

Wespes E, Schulman CC. Haemodynamic study of the effect of vacuum device on human erection. *Int J Impot Res* 1990;2:337.

SURGICAL TREATMENT

Beutler LE, Scott FB, Karacan I et al. Women's satisfaction with partner's penile implant: inflatable versus noninflatable prosthesis. *Urology* 1984;24:552–558.

Carson CC. Penile prostheses. In: Kirby RS, Carson CC, Webster GD, eds. *Impotence: diagnosis and management of erectile dysfunction*. Oxford: Butterworth-Heinemann, 1991:167–176.

Goldstein I. Arterial revascularization procedures. *Semin Urol* 1986;4:252–258.

Goldwasser B, Carson CC, Braun SD, McCann RL. Impotence due to the pelvic steal syndrome: treatment by iliac transluminal angioplasty. *J Urol* 1985;133:860–861.

Kerfoot WW, Carson CC, Donaldson JT, Kliewer MA. Investigation of vascular changes following penile vein ligation. *J Urol* 1994;153:884–887.

Steege JF, Stout AL, Carson CC. Patient satisfaction in Scott and Small-Carrion penile implant recipients: a study of 52 patients. *Arch Sex Behav* 1986;15:393–399.

Woodworth BE, Carson CC, Webster GD. Inflatable penile prosthesis: effect of device modification on function longevity. *Urology* 1991;38:533–536.

Index